MEDITATION AND MINDFULNESS: TECHNIQUES FOR STRESS REDUCTION AND MENTAL CLARITY

OSUNMO TOSIN

ISBN: 9798398260274

DEDICATION

This book is dedicated to all seekers of inner peace, clarity, and well-being.

To those who have embarked on the journey of self-discovery through meditation and mindfulness, may you find solace, strength, and profound transformation in these Pages.

To the countless generations of teachers, gurus, and masters who have shared their wisdom and guided us on the path of mindfulness, we honor your legacy and express our heartfelt gratitude.

To our loved ones, whose support and understanding have been a constant source of inspiration, this dedication is a testament to the love and connection that sustain us on our journey.

And finally, to every reader who has picked up this book, may it serve as a guiding light on your path towards stress reduction, mental clarity, and a life filled with peace, joy, and purpose.

May the wisdom and practices shared within these pages bring you closer to the essence of who you truly are and help you navigate the complexities of life with grace and mindfulness.

With deepest appreciation,

Osunmo Tosin

CONTENTS

TABLE OF CONTENT

INTRODUCTION

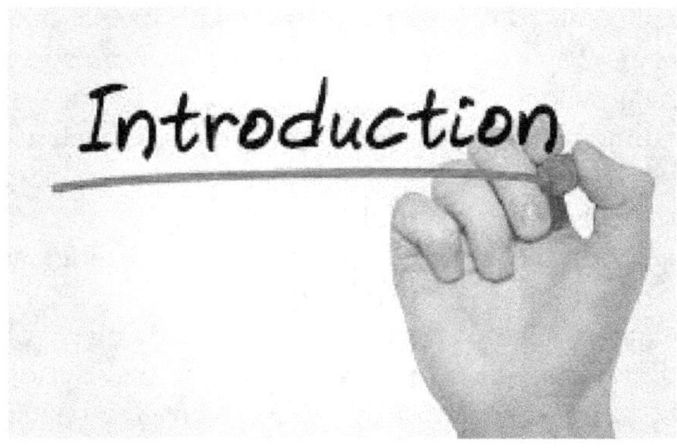

Welcome to "Meditation and Mindfulness: Techniques for Stress Reduction and Mental Clarity." In today's fast-paced and demanding world, it has become increasingly crucial to prioritise our mental well-being. This eBook aims to guide you on a transformative journey towards inner peace, stress reduction, and enhanced mental clarity through the practices of meditation and mindfulness.

A. The Importance of Mental Well-Being: Now more than ever, taking care of our mental health is essential for overall well-being. Our mental state influences every aspect of our lives, from our relationships and work performance to our physical health. By prioritising mental well-being, we can experience greater joy, fulfilment, and resilience in the face of life's challenges.

B. Understanding Stress and Its Impact: Stress has become a pervasive part of our daily lives, affecting us physically, mentally, and emotionally. It can lead to burnout, anxiety, and various health issues. Understanding the impact of stress empowers us to take proactive steps to mitigate its negative effects. Through meditation and mindfulness practices, we can cultivate a calmer state of mind, reduce stress, and improve our overall quality of life.

C. Overview of Meditation and Mindfulness: Meditation and mindfulness have gained significant recognition for their profound impact on mental well-being. These practices involve training our minds to be present, focused, and aware of our thoughts, feelings, and sensations. By incorporating meditation and mindfulness into our lives, we can tap into a deep well of inner peace, clarity, and self-awareness. Throughout this eBook, we will explore various aspects of meditation and mindfulness, providing you with the tools and techniques to embark on your personal journey of self-discovery and transformation. Here's a sneak peek into what lies ahead:

In Chapter II, we will delve into the benefits of meditation and mindfulness, including stress reduction, emotional regulation, improved focus, and enhanced self-awareness.

Chapter III will guide you on getting started with meditation, from setting up your meditation space to establishing a regular practice, overcoming common challenges along the way.

Chapter IV explores different meditation techniques such as mindfulness, loving-kindness, transcendental, guided visualisation, walking, and mantra meditation. Deepening your mindfulness practice is the focus of Chapter V, which covers body scan meditation, mindful eating and drinking, incorporating mindfulness into movement and yoga, and integrating mindfulness into your daily activities. Overcoming obstacles and maintaining consistency in your practice are addressed in Chapter VI, offering insights on dealing with restlessness, managing impatience, finding motivation, and dispelling common myths about meditation.

Chapter VII takes you into the realm of advanced meditation techniques, including breathwork, loving-kindness and compassion practices, insight meditation, and sound and mantra meditation. Integrating mindfulness into various aspects of your life is explored in Chapter VIII, with a particular emphasis on mindful communication, eating, relationships, and work. Chapter IX focuses on nurturing a lifelong meditation practice, with guidance on cultivating gratitude, sustaining motivation, seeking community and support, and continuing personal growth and exploration. Finally, in Chapter X, we wrap up our journey with reflections on the transformative power of meditation and mindfulness, embracing a mindful lifestyle, and offering final words of encouragement. Are you ready to embark on this transformative journey towards stress reduction, mental clarity, and inner peace? Let's begin exploring the remarkable practices of meditation and mindfulness together.

BENEFITS OF MEDITATION AND MINDFULNESS

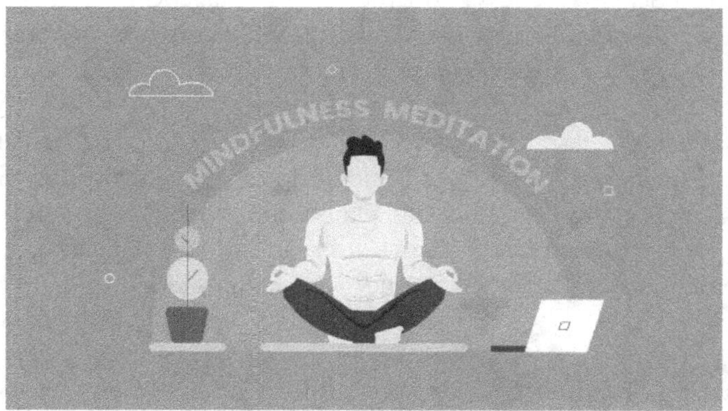

In this chapter, we will explore the remarkable benefits that meditation and mindfulness practices can bring to your life. As you embark on this journey of self-discovery and inner growth, you will discover how these practices can profoundly impact your well-being, providing you with tools to reduce stress, enhance focus, cultivate self-awareness, and embrace mindfulness in your everyday life.

A. Stress Reduction and Emotional Regulation:
In our fast-paced and demanding world, stress has become a common experience for many. Through meditation and mindfulness, you can learn to navigate the challenges of life with greater ease. These practices offer a sanctuary of calm amidst the chaos, allowing you to observe and regulate your emotions effectively. By developing the ability to detach from stressful thoughts and sensations, you can reduce the harmful effects of stress and cultivate a greater sense of inner peace and emotional well-being.

B. Improved Focus and Concentration:
In a world filled with distractions, maintaining focus and concentration has become increasingly challenging. Meditation and mindfulness provide powerful tools to sharpen your attention and improve your ability to

concentrate. By training your mind to anchor itself in the present moment, you develop the capacity to stay focused on tasks and experiences, leading to increased productivity and efficiency. With improved focus, you can fully engage in the present moment, unlocking deeper levels of understanding and creativity.

C. Enhanced Self-Awareness and Emotional Intelligence:
Meditation and mindfulness practices foster self-awareness, inviting you to explore the depths of your own mind, emotions, and experiences. By cultivating a non-judgmental and compassionate attitude towards yourself, you can develop a clearer understanding of your thoughts, beliefs, and reactions. This heightened self-awareness allows you to make conscious choices aligned with your values and goals. Additionally, as you deepen your self-awareness, you naturally enhance your emotional intelligence, leading to more meaningful and authentic connections with others.

D. Cultivating Mindfulness in Everyday Life:
While meditation forms the foundation, the true essence of these practices lies in integrating mindfulness into every aspect of your life. Mindfulness involves bringing a non-judgmental awareness to the present moment, fully engaging with your experiences and cultivating a state of presence. By embracing mindfulness in your daily activities, such as eating, walking, or communicating, you can infuse each moment with intention, gratitude, and a sense of wonder. Mindfulness enables you to live more fully, fostering a deep appreciation for the beauty and richness of everyday life.

Through the practice of meditation and mindfulness, you have the opportunity to experience a transformative shift in your well-being. In the following chapters, we will delve deeper into the practical techniques and exercises that will help you harness these benefits in your own life, empowering you to reduce stress, improve focus, cultivate self-awareness, and embrace mindfulness as a way of living.

GETTING STARTED WITH MEDITATION

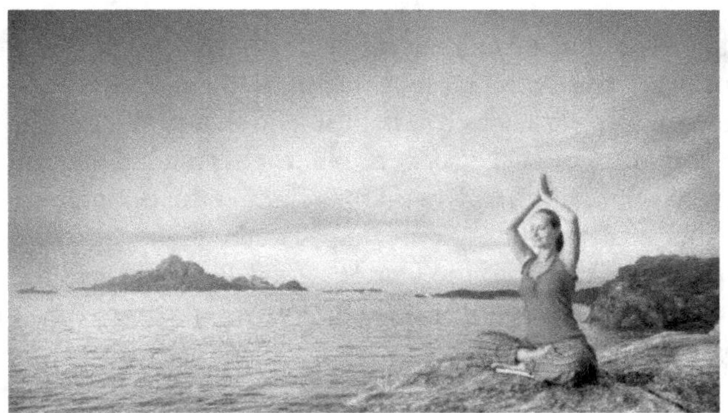

In this chapter, we will explore the foundational elements of starting a meditation practice. Whether you are new to meditation or looking to deepen your existing practice, this chapter will provide you with practical guidance and insights to establish a strong foundation for your journey toward stress reduction and mental clarity.

A. Setting Up Your Meditation Space:
Creating a dedicated meditation space can greatly enhance your practice. We will explore the importance of finding a quiet and comfortable area, free from distractions, where you can retreat and cultivate a sense of tranquillity. You will learn how to arrange your meditation space with meaningful objects, such as cushions, candles, or inspiring images, to create an environment conducive to mindfulness and reflection.

B. Basic Meditation Postures and Breathing Techniques:
Proper posture and breathing techniques play a vital role in meditation. We will explore various meditation postures, such as sitting, kneeling, or even lying down, and discover the importance of aligning your body for optimal comfort and stability. Additionally, we will delve into different breathing techniques that can help you relax, focus your mind, and enter a state of deep meditation.

C. Common Challenges and How to Overcome Them:

Starting a meditation practice can come with its own set of challenges. We will address common obstacles that practitioners often encounter, such as restlessness, difficulty quieting the mind, and physical discomfort. You will learn practical strategies and techniques to overcome these challenges, including gentle mental and physical adjustments, guided imagery, and the power of self-compassion.

D. Establishing a Regular Meditation Practice:
Consistency is key to reaping the benefits of meditation. In this section, we will explore effective strategies to establish and maintain a regular meditation routine. You will discover how to integrate meditation seamlessly into your daily life, whether it's finding the optimal time for your practice, setting realistic goals, or creating accountability structures that support your commitment to meditation. We will also discuss the importance of patience and self-acceptance as you navigate the journey of establishing a regular meditation practice.

By understanding the fundamentals of setting up your meditation space, mastering basic postures and breathing techniques, overcoming common challenges, and establishing a regular practice, you will lay a strong foundation for your meditation journey. These essential aspects will provide you with the tools and support necessary to cultivate mindfulness, reduce stress, and enhance mental clarity.

In the next chapter, we will delve into different meditation techniques, exploring the diverse methods available to you as you deepen your practice and discover what resonates most with your unique needs and preferences.

DIFFERENT MEDITATION TECHNIQUES

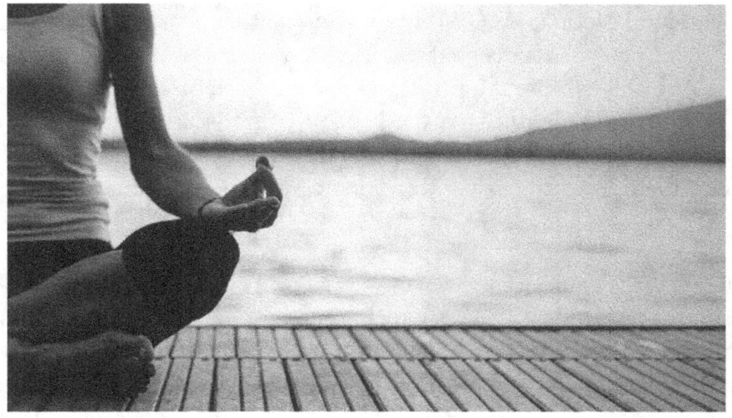

In this chapter, we will explore a variety of meditation techniques that can enrich your practice and deepen your connection with yourself and the present moment. Each technique offers a unique approach to meditation, allowing you to explore different aspects of your mind, emotions, and inner experiences. By experimenting with these techniques, you will discover the ones that resonate most with you and enhance your journey towards stress reduction and mental clarity.

A. Mindfulness Meditation:
Mindfulness meditation is a cornerstone practice that cultivates present-moment awareness without judgement. We will delve into the foundations of mindfulness meditation, including focusing on the breath, observing bodily sensations, and embracing the flow of thoughts and emotions. Through mindfulness meditation, you will develop the ability to stay grounded in the present moment, observing your experiences with openness and curiosity.

B. Loving-Kindness Meditation:
Loving-kindness meditation, also known as Metta meditation, involves generating feelings of love, compassion, and goodwill towards yourself and

others. We will explore the practice of sending loving-kindness to yourself, loved ones, neutral individuals, and even difficult people. This practice cultivates empathy, compassion, and a deep sense of interconnectedness, fostering emotional well-being and nurturing positive relationships.

C. Transcendental Meditation:

Transcendental Meditation (TM) is a technique that involves repeating a mantra silently to access deep states of relaxation and transcend ordinary thinking. We will explore the principles and practice of TM, including the use of personalised mantras and the process of transcending thoughts to reach a state of deep inner stillness. This technique is known for its calming effects on the mind and body, promoting clarity and rejuvenation.

D. Guided Visualization:

Guided visualisation is a powerful technique that harnesses the imagination to create vivid mental images and scenes. We will explore how guided visualisation can be used to promote relaxation, reduce stress, and enhance overall well-being. Through guided imagery, you can create a sanctuary of tranquillity within your mind, allowing you to tap into your inner resources and cultivate a positive mindset.

E. Walking Meditation:

Walking meditation offers a dynamic and embodied approach to mindfulness practice. We will guide you through the process of walking meditation, where you bring focused awareness to the sensations of walking, the movement of your body, and the environment around you. Walking meditation allows you to integrate mindfulness into your everyday activities, fostering a deep connection with the present moment and the world around you.

F. Mantra Meditation:

Mantra meditation involves the repetition of a sacred word or phrase, known as a mantra, to quiet the mind and deepen concentration. We will explore different mantras and guide you in incorporating mantra meditation into your practice. The rhythmic repetition of a mantra can help still the mind, induce relaxation, and foster a sense of inner peace and spiritual connection.

By exploring these diverse meditation techniques, you will expand your repertoire of practices, enabling you to choose the ones that resonate most with you and bring you closer to your goals of stress reduction, mental clarity, and overall well-being. As we continue this journey, you will have the opportunity to integrate these techniques into your daily life and explore their profound effects on your inner landscape.

DEEPENING YOUR MINDFULNESS PRACTICE

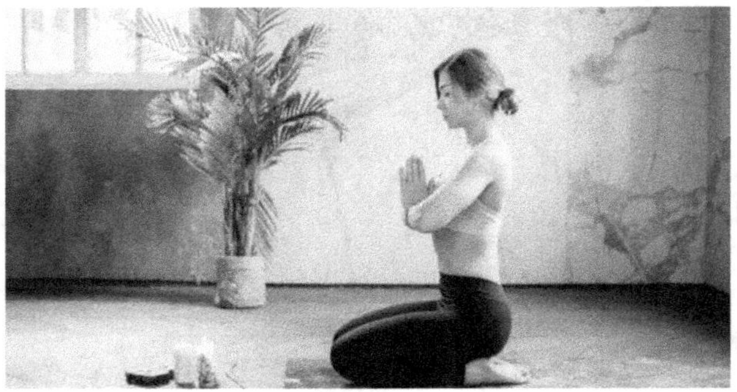

In this chapter, we will delve deeper into the practice of mindfulness, exploring various techniques that allow you to cultivate a deeper sense of presence and awareness in different aspects of your life. By integrating mindfulness into your daily activities, you can infuse each moment with intention, gratitude, and a heightened state of mindfulness.

A. Body Scan Meditation:
The body scan meditation is a powerful technique that involves systematically directing your attention to different parts of your body, bringing a gentle awareness to physical sensations and promoting a deep sense of relaxation. We will guide you through the practice of body scan meditation, allowing you to develop a profound connection with your body, release tension, and enhance body-mind awareness.

B. Mindful Eating and Drinking:
Eating and drinking are everyday activities that often go unnoticed. Mindful eating and drinking involve bringing a non-judgmental and curious awareness to the experience of nourishing your body. We will explore techniques to slow down, savour each bite or sip, and fully engage your senses during mealtimes. By practising mindful eating and drinking, you can cultivate a healthier relationship with food, enhance digestion, and foster a deeper appreciation for the nourishment it provides.

C. Mindful Movement and Yoga:
Movement can be a powerful gateway to mindfulness. We will explore the integration of mindfulness into physical activities, including yoga and mindful movement practices. By combining gentle movements with focused attention on the breath and sensations in the body, you can cultivate a state of embodied awareness, promoting flexibility, strength, and a deeper connection between the mind and body.

D. Incorporating Mindfulness into Daily Activities:
Mindfulness is not limited to formal meditation sessions—it can be integrated into your daily life. We will explore ways to infuse mindfulness into your daily activities, such as brushing your teeth, showering, or commuting. By bringing a mindful presence to these routine activities, you can transform them into opportunities for self-care, relaxation, and heightened awareness. We will provide practical tips and exercises to support you in incorporating mindfulness into various aspects of your day.

By deepening your mindfulness practice through body scan meditation, mindful eating and drinking, mindful movement, and infusing mindfulness into daily activities, you will cultivate a greater sense of presence, gratitude, and self-awareness. These practices will support you in embodying mindfulness as a way of being, transforming your relationship with yourself, others, and the world around you.

OVERCOMING OBSTACLES AND MAINTAINING CONSISTENCY

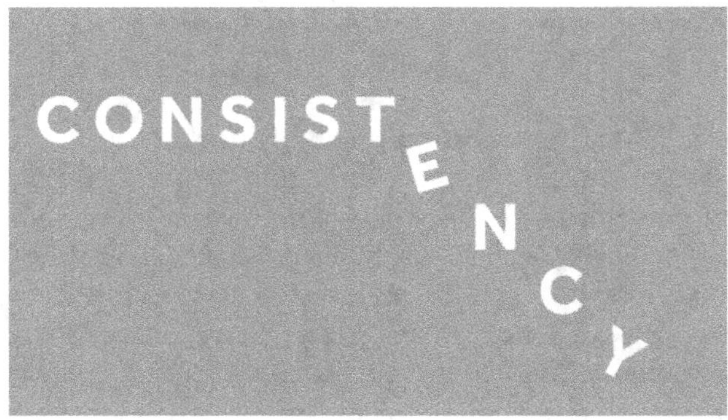

In this chapter, we will explore common challenges that may arise during your meditation and mindfulness practice. By understanding these obstacles and learning effective strategies to overcome them, you can sustain a consistent practice and experience the long-term benefits of meditation and mindfulness.

A Dealing with Restlessness and Monkey Mind:
Restlessness and a wandering mind are common experiences during meditation. We will discuss techniques to navigate restlessness, including bringing gentle awareness back to the present moment, utilising anchor points such as the breath or body sensations, and cultivating patience and acceptance. By developing a compassionate approach towards restlessness and the "monkey mind," you can foster a calmer and more focused state of being.

B. Managing Impatience and Frustration:
Impatience and frustration can arise when progress in your meditation practice feels slow or when expectations are not met. We will explore strategies to manage these emotions, such as practising self-compassion, adjusting expectations, and embracing the process rather than solely focusing on outcomes. By cultivating patience and a non-judgmental attitude towards your practice, you can navigate these challenging emotions and maintain a sense of motivation and dedication.

C. Finding Motivation and Accountability:
Sustaining motivation is crucial for maintaining a consistent meditation
practice. We will discuss ways to cultivate and reignite motivation, such as
clarifying your intentions, setting realistic goals, and finding inspiration
from teachers, books, or meditation communities. Additionally, we will
explore the importance of accountability and how to establish support
systems, whether through meditation groups, meditation apps, or personal
commitments, to help you stay on track with your practice.

D. Overcoming Meditation Myths and Misconceptions:
There are various myths and misconceptions surrounding meditation that
can hinder your progress or discourage you from practising. We will debunk
these myths and provide accurate information to dispel common
misconceptions. By gaining a clear understanding of meditation, you can
approach your practice with an open mind, free from unrealistic
expectations or unnecessary concerns.

By addressing these obstacles and learning effective strategies to overcome
them, you will build resilience, sustain motivation, and maintain a consistent
meditation and mindfulness practice. Embracing the challenges and
dispelling myths will allow you to experience the transformative effects of
meditation and mindfulness more fully, leading to increased stress
reduction, mental clarity, and overall well-being.

ADVANCED MEDITATION TECHNIQUES

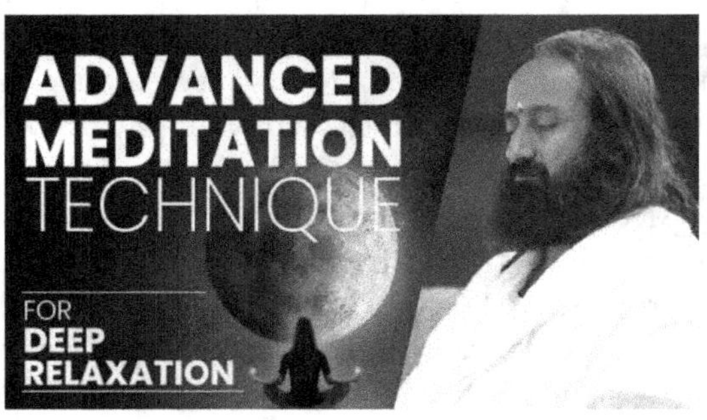

In this chapter, we will explore advanced meditation techniques that can deepen your practice and bring about profound transformative experiences. These techniques go beyond the basics and offer new avenues for self-exploration, inner growth, and spiritual development. By incorporating these advanced techniques into your meditation repertoire, you can further enhance your journey towards stress reduction, mental clarity, and overall well-being.

A. Breathwork and Pranayama:
Breathwork and pranayama involve conscious control and manipulation of the breath to influence the mind and energy flow within the body. We will explore various pranayama techniques, including alternate nostril breathing, deep belly breathing, and breath retention practices. By harnessing the power of the breath, you can cultivate relaxation, balance energy, and deepen your meditation practice.

B. Loving-Kindness and Compassion Practices:
Loving-kindness and compassion practices extend beyond the boundaries of self and embrace all beings with boundless love, care, and empathy. We will guide you through advanced techniques for generating loving-kindness and compassion towards yourself, loved ones, challenging individuals, and all sentient beings. By cultivating these qualities, you can open your heart, dissolve barriers, and experience a profound sense of interconnectedness and well-being.

C. Insight Meditation and Vipassana:
Insight meditation, also known as Vipassana, is a practice of developing clear insight into the nature of reality and the impermanence of all

phenomena. We will explore techniques to cultivate mindfulness and investigate the nature of our thoughts, emotions, and sensory experiences. Through insight meditation, you can develop wisdom, deepen self-understanding, and transcend the illusions of the ego.

D. Sound and Mantra Meditation:
Sound and mantra meditation involve using specific sounds or repetitive phrases to focus the mind and access deeper states of consciousness. We will explore techniques such as chanting, toning, or using sacred sounds to facilitate relaxation, concentration, and spiritual connection. By harnessing the power of sound, you can attune your mind and body to higher frequencies and tap into profound states of inner stillness and harmony.

By incorporating these advanced meditation techniques into your practice, you can expand your horizons, deepen your connection with yourself, and embark on a journey of self-transformation and spiritual growth. Remember, these techniques require patience, dedication, and a willingness to explore new territories of the mind. Embrace the possibilities they offer, and allow them to enrich your meditation practice and your life as a whole.

INTEGRATING MINDFULNESS INTO DAILY LIFE

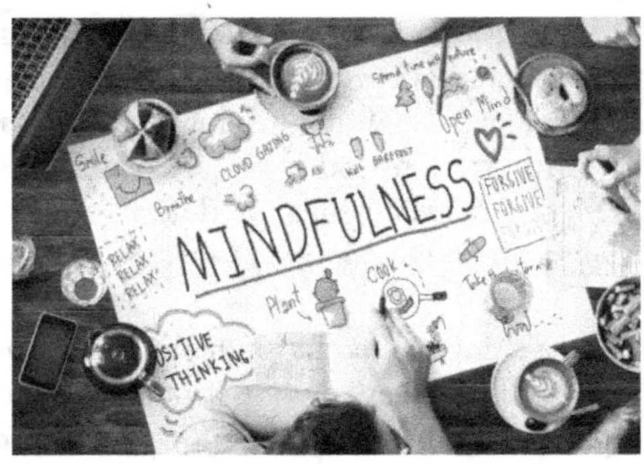

In this chapter, we will explore how to bring the benefits of mindfulness off the meditation cushion and into various aspects of your daily life. By integrating mindfulness into your everyday activities, you can cultivate a greater sense of presence, connection, and well-being in all your interactions and experiences.

A. Mindful Communication and Deep Listening:
Mindful communication involves being fully present and attentive during conversations, cultivating deep listening skills, and responding with clarity and empathy. We will explore techniques for practising mindful communication, such as mindful listening, non-judgmental observation of thoughts and emotions, and choosing words consciously. By incorporating mindfulness into your communication, you can foster healthier and more meaningful connections with others.

B. Mindful Eating and Nutrition:
Mindful eating involves bringing a heightened sense of awareness and presence to the experience of nourishing your body. We will discuss techniques for practising mindful eating, such as savouring each bite, tuning into hunger and fullness cues, and cultivating gratitude for the food you consume. Additionally, we will explore how to make conscious and nourishing choices when it comes to nutrition, supporting your overall well-being.

C. Mindfulness in Relationships and Social Interactions:

Mindfulness can significantly enhance the quality of your relationships and social interactions. We will explore ways to bring mindfulness into your relationships, including practices such as empathy, compassion, and forgiveness. By cultivating presence, deep listening, and non-reactivity, you can foster greater understanding, connection, and harmony in your interactions with loved ones, colleagues, and acquaintances.

D. Mindfulness at Work and in Professional Life:
Bringing mindfulness into the workplace can improve focus, productivity, and overall well-being. We will discuss strategies for integrating mindfulness into your work life, such as mindful work breaks, mindful goal-setting, and managing stress and conflicts with mindfulness. By applying mindfulness to your professional life, you can enhance creativity, decision-making, and cultivate a more fulfilling and balanced work environment.

By integrating mindfulness into your daily life, you can transform routine activities into opportunities for self-awareness, growth, and deepening connections with others. Mindfulness becomes a way of being, infusing your experiences with presence, gratitude, and compassion. Embrace the potential of mindfulness in all areas of your life and witness the positive ripple effects it has on your overall well-being.

NURTURING A LIFELONG MEDITATION PRACTICE

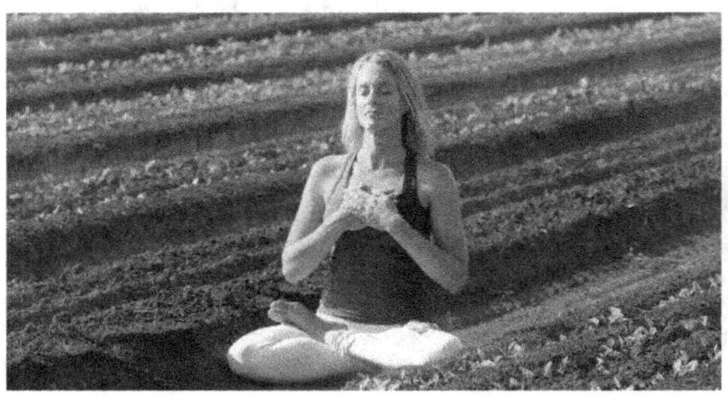

In this chapter, we will explore essential aspects of nurturing a lifelong meditation practice. Building a sustainable and enriching meditation practice goes beyond mastering techniques; it requires cultivating inner qualities, seeking support, and embracing growth and exploration. By incorporating these elements into your journey, you can maintain a vibrant and transformative meditation practice throughout your life.

A. Cultivating Gratitude and Resilience:
Gratitude and resilience are powerful qualities that can support and deepen your meditation practice. We will discuss techniques for cultivating gratitude, such as keeping a gratitude journal and practising appreciation for the present moment. Additionally, we will explore how to develop resilience, bounce back from challenges, and stay committed to your practice even during difficult times. By cultivating these qualities, you can enhance your overall well-being and sustain a positive outlook on your meditation journey.

B. Sustaining Motivation and Consistency:
Motivation and consistency are vital for maintaining a lifelong meditation practice. We will explore strategies for sustaining motivation, including setting meaningful intentions, tracking progress, and celebrating milestones. Additionally, we will discuss practical tips for establishing a consistent meditation routine, overcoming obstacles, and navigating periods of resistance or low motivation. By nurturing motivation and consistency, you can deepen your practice and reap the long-term benefits of meditation.

C. Seeking Community and Support:

Engaging with a community and finding support can greatly enhance your meditation practice. We will discuss the importance of connecting with like-minded individuals, joining meditation groups or retreats, and seeking guidance from experienced practitioners or teachers. Additionally, we will explore the benefits of accountability partners and how they can provide support, inspiration, and a sense of belonging on your meditation journey. By cultivating a supportive network, you can stay inspired, share insights, and learn from others' experiences.

D. Continuing Growth and Exploration:
A lifelong meditation practice is a journey of continuous growth and exploration. We will discuss the importance of embracing curiosity, remaining open to new techniques and perspectives, and expanding your meditation repertoire. Additionally, we will explore how to integrate other complementary practices such as mindfulness-based therapies, bodywork, or creative expressions into your meditation journey. By embracing ongoing growth and exploration, you can deepen your practice, expand your understanding, and continue to evolve on your spiritual path.

By nurturing these aspects of your meditation practice, you can create a strong foundation for a lifelong journey of self-discovery, inner transformation, and spiritual growth. Embrace the qualities of gratitude and resilience, sustain motivation and consistency, seek community and support, and remain open to growth and exploration. Through these practices, your meditation journey can become a profound and fulfilling lifelong path.

CONCLUSION

In this final chapter of "Meditation and Mindfulness: Techniques for Stress Reduction and Mental Clarity," we reflect on the transformative power of meditation and mindfulness, explore the importance of embracing a mindful lifestyle, and offer final words of encouragement to support you on your journey.

A. The Transformative Power of Meditation and Mindfulness:
Throughout this book, we have delved into the numerous benefits that meditation and mindfulness can bring to your life. We have explored how these practices can reduce stress, enhance mental clarity, improve focus and concentration, and cultivate emotional regulation and self-awareness. It is essential to acknowledge that the power of meditation and mindfulness extends beyond these tangible benefits. Through consistent practice, you have the opportunity to connect with your inner self, tap into your innate wisdom, and experience profound transformation on a deeper level. By cultivating mindfulness, you open the door to greater self-discovery, compassion, and inner peace.

B. Embracing a Mindful Lifestyle:
Beyond formal meditation sessions, embracing a mindful lifestyle involves integrating the principles of mindfulness into every aspect of your life. It means bringing awareness, presence, and compassion to your interactions, activities, and choices. By applying mindfulness to your communication, relationships, work, and daily routines, you can create a more fulfilling and harmonious life. Embracing a mindful lifestyle allows you to live with intention, appreciate the present moment, and navigate life's challenges with greater resilience and equanimity.

C. Final Words of Encouragement:
As you conclude this book and continue your meditation and mindfulness journey, remember that it is a lifelong practice. Be patient with yourself, as progress may unfold gradually. Embrace the moments of stillness and insight that arise during meditation, and carry their wisdom into your daily life. Embrace the imperfections and challenges that may arise along the way, knowing that they are opportunities for growth and learning. Remember that your practice is unique to you, and it may evolve and adapt as you do. Trust in the process, and be gentle and compassionate with yourself throughout the journey.

May your meditation and mindfulness practice continue to be a source of peace, clarity, and self-discovery. Embrace the transformative power of these practices, weave mindfulness into the fabric of your life, and let them guide you towards a deeper understanding of yourself and the world around you. Remember that every moment offers an opportunity for presence and mindfulness. Embrace this moment, and let it be the starting point for a lifetime of growth and well-being.

Wishing you joy, peace, and fulfilment on your meditation and mindfulness journey.

End of "Meditation and Mindfulness: Techniques for Stress Reduction and Mental Clarity."

ABOUT THE AUTHOR

Osunmo Tosin The author of "Meditation and Mindfulness: Techniques for Stress Reduction and Mental Clarity," is a passionate advocate for personal growth, well-being, and mindfulness. With a deep-rooted interest in exploring the depths of the human mind and spirit, Osunmo Tosin has dedicated their life to understanding and sharing the transformative power of meditation and mindfulness.

Having personally experienced the positive impact of these practices, Osunmo Tosin brings a genuine and empathetic approach to their writing. With a background in psychology and extensive training in various meditation modalities, they possess a wealth of knowledge and expertise in guiding others towards inner peace and clarity.

Combining their academic insights with practical wisdom gained from years of personal practice, Osunmo Tosin has crafted this book to provide readers with a comprehensive roadmap to harness the benefits of meditation and mindfulness in their daily lives. Their writing is characterized by a warm and accessible style, making complex concepts easily understandable for readers of all backgrounds.

As an experienced meditation teacher and mindfulness coach, Osunmo Tosin has had the privilege of witnessing the transformative journeys of countless individuals. Through their work, they strive to inspire and empower others to cultivate a more mindful and fulfilling life, filled with greater self-awareness, emotional balance, and resilience.

When not writing or teaching, Osunmo Tosin enjoys immersing themselves in nature, practicing yoga, and exploring new avenues for personal growth. They firmly believe that the journey of self-discovery is a lifelong adventure, and they continue to expand their knowledge and understanding through ongoing study and exploration.

Through their book, "Meditation and Mindfulness: Techniques for Stress Reduction and Mental Clarity," Osunmo Tosin shares their passion, insights, and practical guidance to help readers embark on their own transformative journey towards inner peace and well-being. Their sincere hope is that this book will serve as a valuable resource and companion on the path to a more mindful and purposeful life.